Soup Recipes

Top 30 Recipes: European Soups, 5 ingredients Soups and Broth, Garlic, Tomato and Egg Soups, Kids Recipes

Table of Content

Introduction

Soup is a quick, hot meal that offers plenty of health benefits. You can throw a variety of ingredients into a slow cooker in the morning before you leave for work or school and return home to a delicious meal in the evening. The healthiest soups include fresh, low-fat ingredients and a minimum of salt and extra fat.

The American Heart Association recommends adults consume 8 or more servings of fruits and vegetables every day. That's 4 cups. Soups can contribute to that total! Almost any vegetable lends itself to use in soup. Vegetables in soup contain many vitamins, such as A and C, calcium and vitamin D.

Soups made with beans and lean meats such as fish provide lean protein. Beans also give you fiber. Tomatoes are a good source of lycopene, an antioxidant that may help reduce the risk of cancer.

Most soups, if made with lean meat, are low in fat, making them a good choice for anyone concerned about fat in his diet.

Here are top reasons why you should eat soup:

1. Soup is a quick meal.

It is easy to make. With only a few ingredients, one can make a bowl of hearty soup for a cold evening.

2. Soup is good for the health.

Perhaps the easiest way to add vegetables to your daily meals is to make and eat soup. You can make several bowls of soup filled with fruits and veggies each day and you'll be filled. Eating vegetables is part of a healthy diet so veggie soups are highly recommended.

3. Soup can help you lose weight.

Soups are slimming. Of course, that is if you strictly follow a weight-loss plan and exercise more. A bowl of soup packs minimal calorie but is very nutritious.

4. Soup makes you feel full.

Soup fills you up because it stretches the stomach. You easily feel full so it's ideal to eat soup at the beginning of every meal.

5. Soup is affordable to make.

Making soup won't require a lot of money. Buy some vegetables and fruits, broth or water, and you can easily make a batch enough to feed the entire family. For a small cost, you can make a lot of people feel full!

5 ingredients Soups and Broth

Beefy Corn and Black Bean Chili

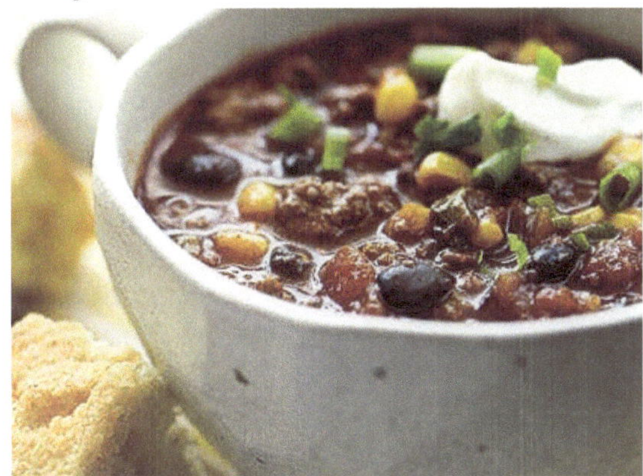

Serves: 6   Calories: 193

Preparation Time: 20 minutes

Ingredients

- 1 pound ground round
- 2 teaspoons salt-free chili powder blend
- 1 (14-ounce) package frozen seasoned corn and black beans
- 1 (14-ounce) can fat-free, less-sodium beef broth
- 1 (15-ounce) can seasoned tomato sauce for chili

Method

1. Combine beef and chili powder blend in a large Dutch oven. Cook 6 minutes over medium-high heat or until beef is browned, stirring to crumble. Drain and return to pan.
2. Stir in frozen corn mixture, broth, and tomato sauce; bring to a boil. Cover, reduce heat, and simmer 10 minutes.
3. Uncover and simmer 5 minutes, stirring occasionally.
4. Ladle chili into bowls.
5. Top each serving with sour cream and onions, if desired.

Posole

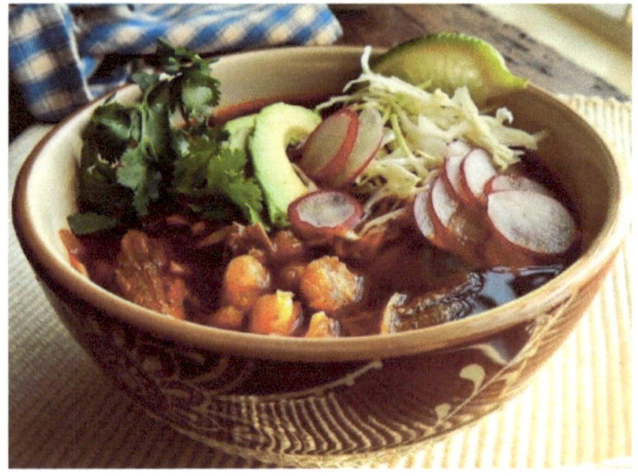

Serves: 6   Calories: 233

Preparation Time: 20 minutes

Ingredients

- 1 (1-pound) pork tenderloin, trimmed and cut into bite-sized pieces
- 2 teaspoons salt-free Southwest chipotle seasoning blend
- 1 (15.5-ounce) can white hominy, undrained
- 1 (14.5-ounce) can Mexican-style stewed tomatoes with jalapeno peppers and spices, undrained
- 1/4 cup chopped fresh cilantro

Method

1. Heat a large saucepan over medium-high heat. Coat pan with cooking spray.
2. Sprinkle pork evenly with chipotle seasoning blend; coat evenly with cooking spray.
3. Add pork to pan; cook 4 minutes or until browned. Stir in hominy, tomatoes, and 1 cup water.
4. Bring to a boil; cover, reduce heat, and simmer 20 minutes or until pork is tender. Stir in cilantro.

Spicy Poblano and Corn Soup

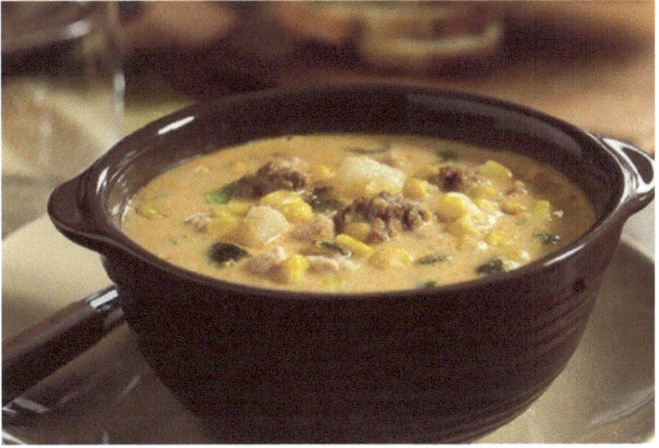

Serves: 6   Calories: 239

Preparation Time: 10 minutes

Ingredients

- 1 (16-ounce) package frozen baby gold and white corn, thawed and divided
- 2 cups fat-free milk, divided
- 4 poblano chiles, seeded and chopped (about 1 pound)
- 1 cup refrigerated prechopped onion
- 1/2 cup (2 ounces) reduced-fat shredded sharp cheddar cheese

Method

1. Place 1 cup corn and 1 1/2 cups milk in a Dutch oven. Bring mixture to a boil over medium heat.
2. Combine chopped chile, onion, and 1 tablespoon water in a microwave-safe bowl. Cover and microwave at HIGH 4 minutes.
3. Meanwhile, place 2 cups corn and 1/2 cup milk in a blender; process until smooth.
4. Add pureed mixture to corn mixture in pan. Stir in chile mixture and salt, and cook 6 minutes over medium heat.
5. Ladle soup into bowls, and top each serving with 2 tablespoons cheddar cheese.

Southwestern Chicken and White Bean Soup

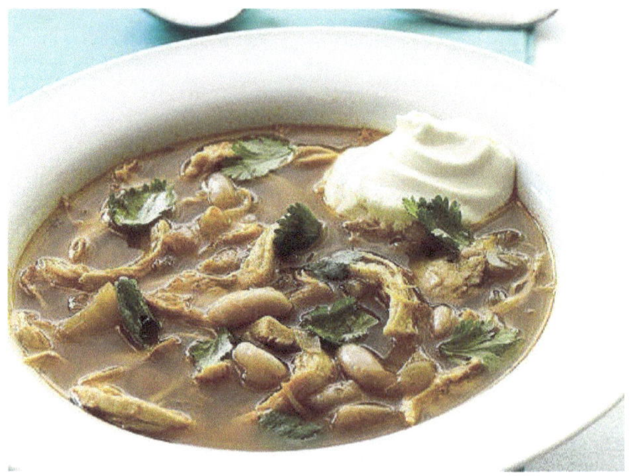

Serves: 4   Calories: 134

Preparation Time: 12 minutes

Ingredients

- 2 cups shredded cooked chicken breast
- 1 tablespoon 40%-less-sodium taco seasoning
- 2 (14-ounce) cans fat-free, less-sodium chicken broth
- 1 (16-ounce) can cannellini beans or other white beans, rinsed and drained
- 1/2 cup green salsa

Method

1. Combine chicken and taco seasoning; toss well to coat. Heat a large saucepan over medium-high heat. Coat pan with cooking spray.
2. Add chicken; cook for 2 minutes or until chicken is lightly browned.
3. Add broth, scraping pan to loosen browned bits.
4. Place beans in a small bowl; mash until only a few whole beans remain.
5. Add beans and salsa to pan, stirring well. Bring to a boil.
6. Reduce heat; simmer 10 minutes or until slightly thick.
7. Serve with sour cream and cilantro, if desired.

Chicken-Escarole Soup

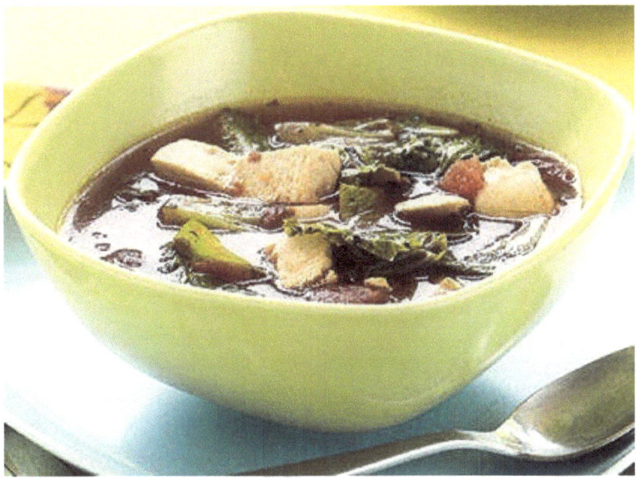

Serves: 4   Calories: 118

Preparation Time: 10 minutes

Ingredients

- 1 (14 1/2-ounce) can Italian-style stewed tomatoes, undrained and chopped
- 1 (14-ounce) can fat-free, less-sodium chicken broth
- 1 cup chopped cooked chicken breast
- 2 cups coarsely chopped escarole (about 1 small head)
- 2 teaspoons extra-virgin olive oil

Method

1. Combine tomatoes and broth in a large saucepan.
2. Cover and bring to a boil over high heat.
3. Reduce heat to low; simmer 5 minutes.
4. Add chicken, escarole, and oil; cook 5 minutes.

European Soups Recipes

Tea-Scented Pumpkin Soup

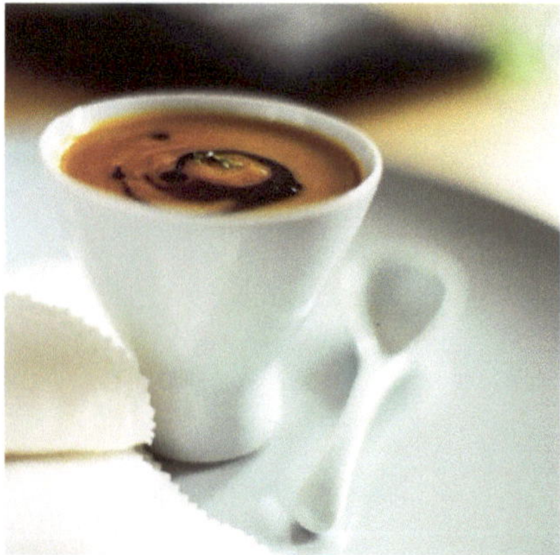

Serves: 8

Cook Time: 30 mins

Ingredients

- One 3-pound sweet pumpkin or kabocha squash—quartered, seeded, peeled and cut into 2-inch pieces
- 6 cups chicken stock or vegetable stock
- 1 teaspoon Ceylon tea
- 1/2 cup boiling water
- Salt and freshly ground pepper
- 2 teaspoons vegetable oil
- 2 scallions, green part only, thinly sliced crosswise
- Roasted pumpkinseed oil, for drizzling

Method

1. In a large enameled cast-iron casserole, cover the pumpkin with the stock and bring to a boil. Simmer over moderate heat until the pumpkin is tender, about 35 minutes.
2. In a cup, steep the tea in the boiling water for 5 minutes. Strain the tea.
3. Working in batches, puree the soup in a blender and return it to the casserole. Add the tea and bring to a simmer. Season the soup with salt and pepper.
4. In a small skillet, heat the vegetable oil. Add the scallion greens and cook over high heat until softened, about 30 seconds. Season with salt.

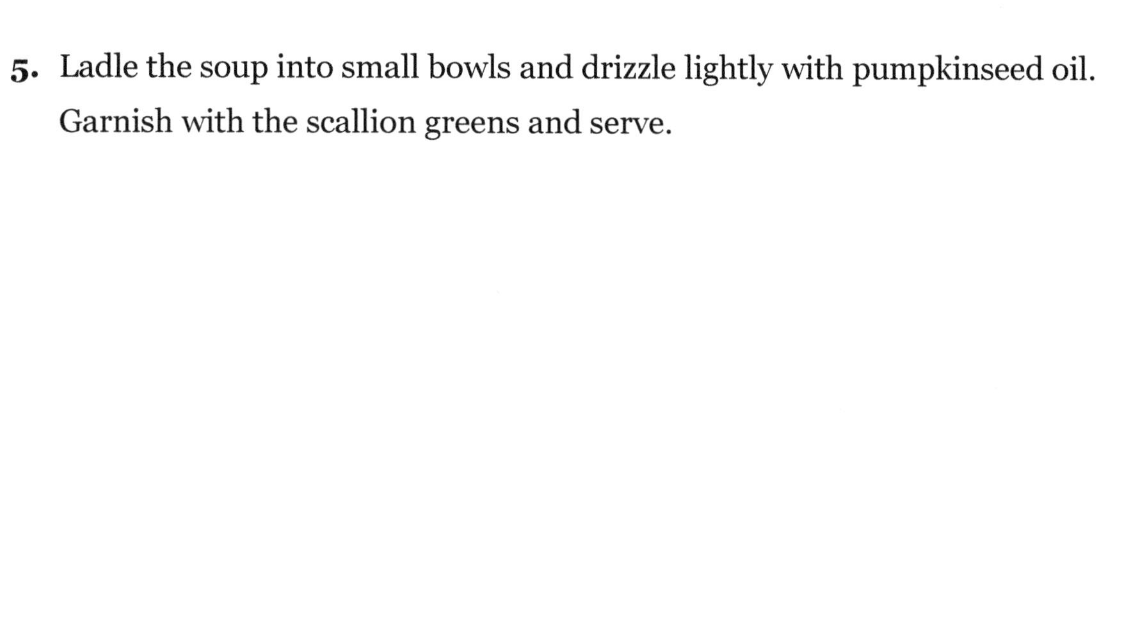

5. Ladle the soup into small bowls and drizzle lightly with pumpkinseed oil. Garnish with the scallion greens and serve.

Chicken And Rice Soup

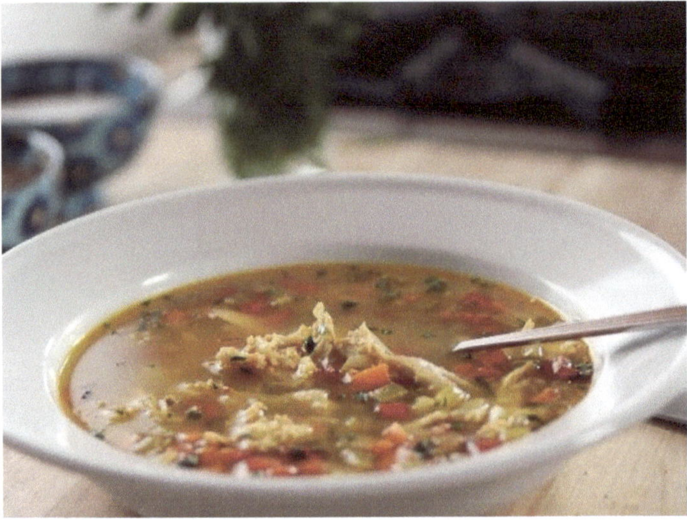

Serves: 4

Cooking Time: 45 minutes

Ingredients

- 8 cups water
- 2 chicken breast halves; skin and fat removed
- 2 whole chicken legs with thighs; skin and fat removed
- 3 carrots, peeled, halved crosswise
- 3 celery stalks, quartered crosswise
- 1 onion, sliced
- 2 teaspoons salt
- 2 garlic cloves, chopped
- 1 bay leaf
- 3/4 cup uncooked long-grain white rice
- Chopped fresh parsley

Method

1. Combine first 9 ingredients in large pot. Bring to boil. Reduce heat, cover and simmer until chicken is cooked through, about 30 minutes.
2. Using slotted spoon, transfer chicken and carrots to platter; cool slightly. Pull chicken meat off bones in bite-size pieces; set aside. Discard bones. Thinly slice carrots and reserve.
3. Strain broth; discard solids in strainer. Pour 1 1/2 cups broth into heavy medium saucepan. Bring to boil. Add rice and bring to boil.
4. Reduce heat to low; cover and cook until broth is absorbed and rice is tender, about 20 minutes.

5. Return remaining broth, chicken pieces and sliced carrots to same large pot. Bring to simmer. Stir in cooked rice.
6. Season soup with salt and pepper. Ladle soup into bowls. Sprinkle with parsley and serve.
7. Enjoy!

Pumpkin and Yellow Split Pea Soup

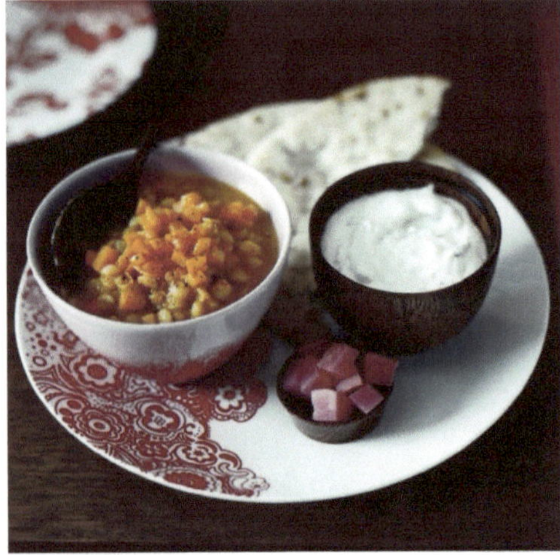

Serves: 12

Cook Time: 25 mins

Ingredients

- 4 tablespoons unsalted butter
- 1 medium red onion, cut into 1/4-inch dice
- 4 garlic cloves, minced
- 1 serrano chile, seeded and minced
- 1 1/2 teaspoons ground cumin
- 1/2 teaspoon cayenne pepper
- 2 cups yellow split peas, soaked in water for 1 hour and drained
- 8 1/2 cups water
- One 15-ounce can unsweetened pumpkin puree
- 3/4 pound fresh sugar pumpkin or butternut squash, peeled and cut into 1/4-inch dice
- 1 1/2 tablespoons fresh lemon juice
- Kosher salt and freshly ground pepper

Method

1. In a large pot, melt the butter. Add the onion, garlic, and chile and cook over moderately high heat until the onion is softened, 4 minutes.
2. Add the cumin and cayenne and cook until fragrant, about 1 minute. Add the split peas and the water, then whisk in the pumpkin puree and bring to a simmer. Cover and cook over moderately low heat, stirring occasionally, until the split peas are tender, about 2 hours.

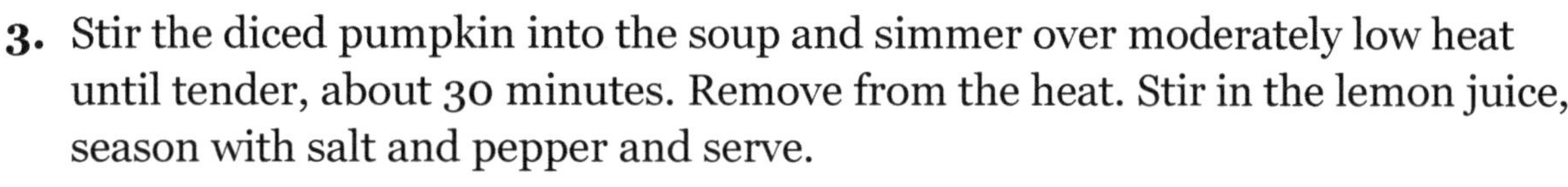

3. Stir the diced pumpkin into the soup and simmer over moderately low heat until tender, about 30 minutes. Remove from the heat. Stir in the lemon juice, season with salt and pepper and serve.

White Bean and Kale Soup

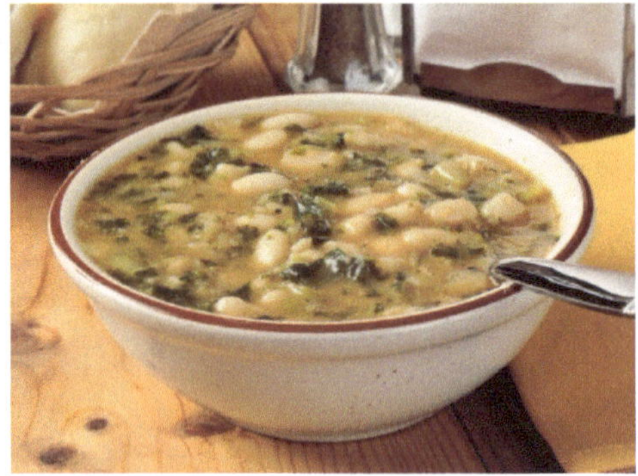

Serves: 4   Calories: 362

Cooking Time: 25 minutes

Ingredients

- 2 tbsp Olive oil
- 1 small Onions
- 30 oz Cannellini Beans
- 4 cup Organic Vegetable Stock
- 2 cup Water
- 2 cup, chopped Kale
- 1 dash Salt
- 1 dash Pepper

Method

1. Heat the oil in a 3 quart saucepan over medium-high heat until shimmering. Add chopped onion and cook until softened, about 5 minutes.
2. Meanwhile, mash one can of beans in a small bowl. Add mashed beans, broth, and water to saucepan. Bring to a boil.
3. Stir in remaining beans (left whole), kale, 1 tsp. Salt, and ¼ tsp. pepper. Reduce heat, partially cover, and simmer about 20 minutes, until kale is tender.
4. Season to taste with additional salt and pepper and serve.

Black Bean Soup

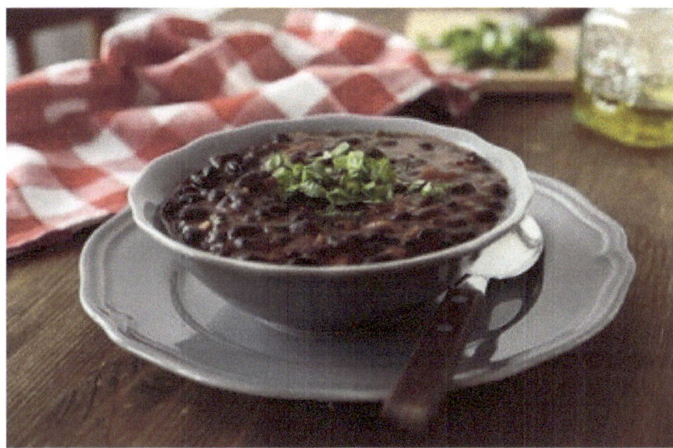

Serves: 1   Calories: approx 350 (without toppings)

Preparation Time: 30 minutes

Ingredients

- ½ tin black beans
- ½ tin canned tomatoes
- ½ onion
- 1 red bell pepper
- 1 clove garlic
- ½ stalk celery
- 1 tsp chilli powder
- ½ carrot
- 1 cup vegetable broth
- 1 tsp fresh or dried oregano, chopped
- 1 tsp olive oil
- Pinch of salt
- Pinch of black pepper
- Your choice of toppings (chopped green onion, fresh herbs, sliced avocado, etc)

Method

1. Dice the onion, carrot, red pepper and celery.
2. Mince or finely chop the garlic.
3. Heat the oil in a large saucepan and add the onion, carrot, garlic, red pepper and celery. Sauté for five minutes.
4. Add the herbs and salt and sauté for another minute or so.

5. Add the vegetable broth and half the beans.

6. In a blender or food processor, blend the tomatoes and remaining beans until smooth.

7. Add the bean and tomato mixture to the soup along with the chilli powder and black pepper.

8. Simmer for fifteen minutes.

9. Top with whatever you prefer and eat while hot.

Pumpkin Soup with Sage and Ham

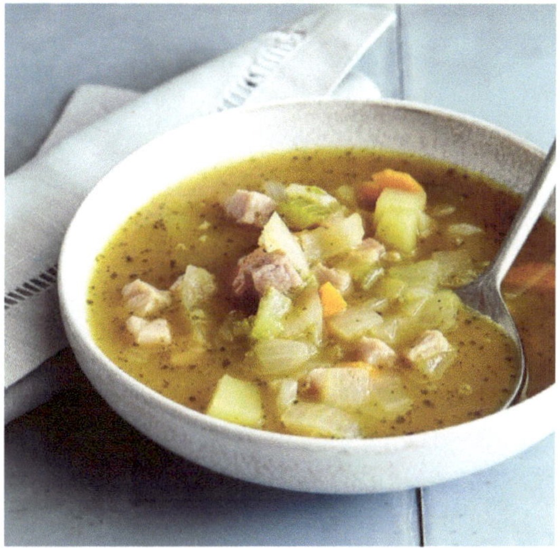

Serves: 4

Cook Time: 25 mins

Ingredients

- 3 tablespoons butter
- 1 onion, chopped
- 1 carrot, chopped
- 1 rib celery, chopped
- 1/2 tart apple, such as Granny Smith, peeled, cored, and cut into 1/2-inch dice
- 2 cups canned pumpkin puree (from one 29-ounce can)
- 1/3 cup dry white wine
- 1 tablespoon dried sage
- 1 bay leaf
- 3 1/2 cups water
- 2 1/2 cups canned low-sodium chicken broth or homemade stock
- 1 1/2 teaspoons salt
- 1/4 teaspoon fresh-ground black pepper
- 1 1/2-pound piece of ham, cut into 1/4-inch dice

Method

1. In a large pot, melt the butter over moderate heat.
2. Add the onion, carrot, celery, and apple and cook, stirring occasionally, until the onion is translucent, about 10 minutes.
3. Stir in the pumpkin puree, wine, sage, and bay leaf.
4. Add the water, broth, salt, and pepper and bring to a simmer. Reduce the heat and simmer, partially covered, for 15 minutes.

5. Add the ham and simmer, uncovered, until the vegetables are tender, about 5 minutes longer. Remove the bay leaf.

Sausage Wild Rice Soup

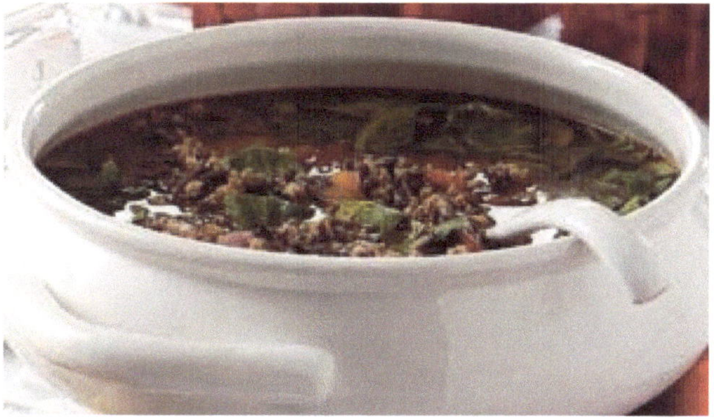

Serves: 13

Cook Time: 60 mins

Ingredients

- 9 cups water, divided
- 1 cup uncooked wild rice
- 2 pounds bulk Italian sausage
- 2 large onions, chopped
- 2 teaspoons olive oil
- 6 garlic cloves, minced
- 3 cartons (32 ounces each) chicken broth
- 1 can (28 ounces) diced tomatoes, undrained
- 1 can (6 ounces) tomato paste
- 2 teaspoons dried basil
- 2 teaspoons dried oregano
- 1 package (6 ounces) fresh baby spinach, coarsely chopped
- 1/2 teaspoon salt
- 1/2 teaspoon pepper

Method

1. In a large saucepan, bring 3 cups water to a boil.
2. Stir in rice. Reduce heat; cover and simmer for 55-60 minutes or until tender.
3. Meanwhile, in a stockpot, cook sausage over medium heat until no longer pink; drain. Remove and set aside.
4. In the same pan, saute onions in oil until tender. Add garlic; cook 1 minute longer. Stir in the broth, tomatoes, tomato paste, basil, oregano and remaining water. Return sausage to the pan. Bring to a boil.
5. Reduce heat; simmer, uncovered, for 20 minutes.
6. Stir in the spinach, salt, pepper and wild rice; heat through.

Italian Sausage Soup

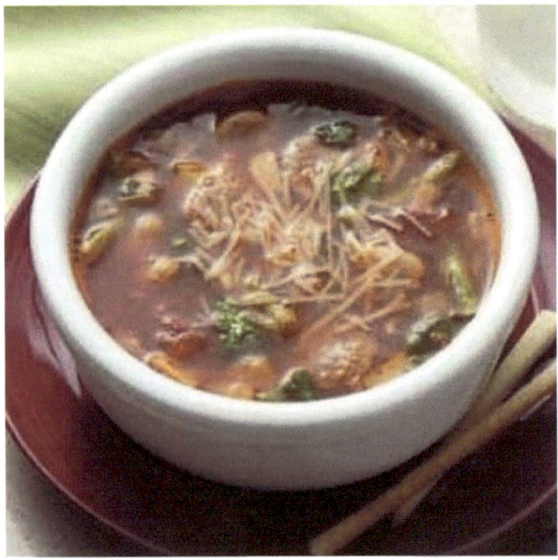

Serves: 8

Cook Time: 45 mins

Ingredients

- 1 can (49-1/2 ounces) chicken broth
- 2 cups cut fresh green beans
- 1 can (15 ounces) cannellini or white kidney beans, rinsed and drained
- 1 can (14-1/2 ounces) Italian diced tomatoes
- 1 cup chopped onion
- 1 cup chopped celery
- 1 cup chopped fennel bulb
- 1 can (6 ounces) tomato paste
- 1 teaspoon dried oregano
- 1/2 teaspoon white pepper
- 5 Italian sausage links
- 1 tablespoon olive oil
- 3 cups coarsely chopped fresh spinach
- Shredded Parmesan cheese, optional

Method

1. In a Dutch oven, combine the first 10 ingredients. Bring to a boil. Reduce heat; cover and simmer for 20 minutes.
2. Meanwhile, in a large skillet, brown sausage in oil over medium heat. Add a small amount of hot water. Cover and cook until sausage is no longer pink;

drain. Cut into 1/4-in. slices and add to soup. Simmer, uncovered, for 15 minutes.

3. Add spinach. Simmer, uncovered, for 5 minutes or until spinach is wilted. Garnish with Parmesan cheese if desired.

Garlic Soups

Garlic Soup with Potatoes and Poached Eggs

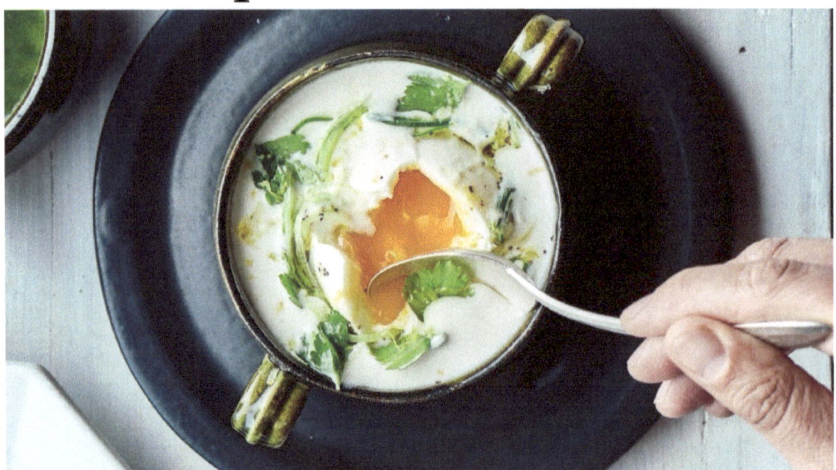

Serves: 4   Calories: 480

Preparation Time: 45 minutes

Ingredients

- 2 tablespoons olive oil, plus more for serving
- 4 tablespoons salted butter, divided
- 3 heads of garlic, cloves peeled
- 1 large leek, halved lengthwise, very thinly sliced, dark green parts reserved separately
- 1 tablespoon thyme leaves
- 1½ pounds Yukon Gold potatoes (about 2 large), peeled, cut into 1-inch pieces
- 4 cups (or more) low-sodium chicken broth
- 2 tablespoons sour cream, room temperature
- Kosher salt
- Freshly ground white or black pepper
- 4 large eggs, room temperature
- 2 tablespoons parsley leaves with tender stems
- Finely grated lemon zest (for serving)

Method

1. Heat 2 Tbsp. oil and 2 Tbsp. butter in a large saucepan over medium. Add garlic, white and pale green parts of leek, and thyme and cook, stirring often, until garlic is softened, about 5 minutes (reduce heat if garlic starts to brown).
2. Add potatoes and 4 cups broth, bring to a simmer, and cook until potatoes are very tender, 25–30 minutes. Let cool slightly, then add creme fraîche.

3. Transfer soup to a blender (or use an immersion blender directly in saucepan) and blend until very smooth; season with salt and pepper. Transfer soup back to saucepan and set aside.

4. Pour water into another large saucepan to come 4 up sides and bring to a boil, then reduce heat so water is at a gentle simmer. Crack an egg into a small bowl, then gently slide egg into water. Repeat with remaining eggs, waiting until whites are opaque before adding the next one (about 30 seconds apart). Poach until whites are set but yolks are still runny, about 3 minutes. Using a slotted spoon, transfer eggs to paper towels as they are done; season with salt and pepper.

5. Heat remaining 2 Tbsp. butter in a medium saucepan over medium. Add reserved dark green parts of leek and 2 Tbsp. water and cook, stirring often, until leeks are softened and very bright green, about 2 minutes. Transfer leek mixture to a platter and top with parsley leaves and lemon zest.

6. Gently reheat reserved soup over medium-low, thinning with more broth if needed; divide among bowls. Carefully place a poached egg and some leek mixture in the center of each bowl of soup and drizzle with oil.

Roasted Garlic Soup With Parmesan

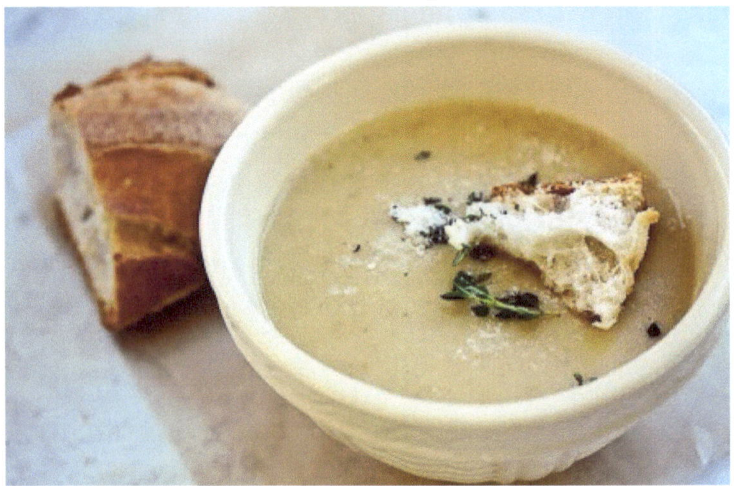

Serves: 4   Calories: 145

Preparation Time: 35 minutes

Ingredients

- 26 cloves roasted garlic (2-3 heads)
- 2 tablespoons olive oil
- 2 tablespoons butter
- 2 1/4 cups sliced onions
- 1 1/2 teaspoons chopped fresh thyme
- 18 cloves garlic, peeled
- 3 1/2 cups chicken stock or 3 1/2 cups vegetable stock
- 1/2 cup whipping cream
- 1/2 cup finely grated parmesan cheese (about 2 ounces)
- 4 lemon wedges

Method

1. Melt butter in heavy large saucepan over medium-high heat; add onions and thyme and cook until onions are translucent, about 6 minutes.
2. Add roasted garlic and 18 raw garlic cloves and cook 3 minutes.
3. Add chicken stock; cover and simmer until garlic is very tender, about 20 minutes.
4. Working in batches, puree soup in blender until smooth.
5. Return soup to saucepan; add cream and bring to simmer.
6. Season with salt and pepper.
7. Divide grated cheese among 4 bowls and ladle soup over.
8. Squeeze juice of 1 lemon wedge into each bowl and serve.

40 Cloves Of Garlic Soup

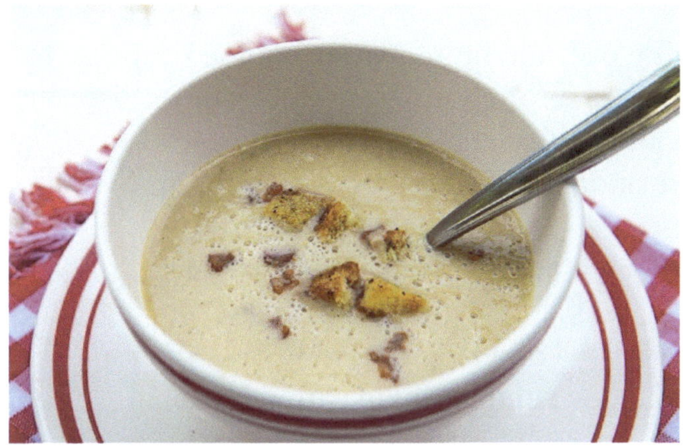

Serves: 4   Calories: 140

Preparation Time: 1 hour 40 minutes

Ingredients

- 25 garlic cloves, unpeeled + 15 garlic cloves, peeled
- 2 tablespoons olive oil
- 2 tablespoons unsalted butter
- 2 1/4 cups sliced onions (about 1 medium onion)
- 1/2 teaspoon dried thyme (or 1 1/2 teaspoons fresh thyme)
- 3 cups vegetable broth
- 1/2 cup heavy whipping cream
- Kosher (coarse) salt and freshly ground pepper
- 1/2 cup shredded Parmesan cheese
- 4 lemon wedges

Method

1. Preheat oven to 350F/175C. Cut the top(s) off of your head(s) of garlic and separate out 25 cloves, making sure each clove has an end chopped off (this will help with squeezing out the roasted garlic later on).
2. Place the 25 cloves in a small glass baking dish, pour the 2 tablespoons of olive oil over the top, and sprinkle with a little salt and pepper. Toss to coat. Cover the baking dish with foil and bake for about 45 minutes, until cloves are light golden brown and very tender. Remove from oven and cool.
3. Squeeze the roasted garlic between your fingertips to release the garlic and discard the peel. Set roasted garlic aside.
4. In a large saucepan, melt the butter over medium heat. Add the onions and thyme; cook until onions are soft and translucent, about 5 minutes. Add both

the roasted garlic and the 15 peeled raw garlic cloves and cook, stirring, for about 3 minutes.

5. Add vegetable stock and, continuing over medium heat, bring the soup just to a boil. Reduce heat and simmer, covered, for about 20 minutes, or until garlic is very tender. Remove from heat and cool slightly.
6. Using an immersion blender or working in batches with a blender, puree soup until smooth.
7. Return soup to pan and stir in heavy whipping cream. Season with salt and pepper, to taste.
8. Sprinkle Parmesan cheese into each bowl and ladle the soup over the top. Squeeze one lemon wedge over each bowl and sprinkle with additional Parmesan if desired.
9. Serve!

Zucchini Garlic Soup

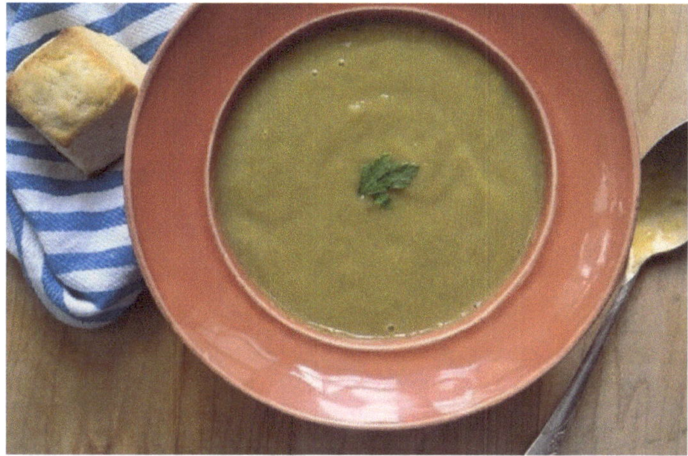

Serves: 4   Calories: 153

Preparation Time: 55 minutes

Ingredients

- 4 tablespoons unsalted butter
- 1 white onion, sliced
- 8 to 9 large cloves garlic, sliced thinly
- 4 medium zucchini, about 1 1/2 pounds
- 4 cups chicken or vegetable broth
- 1/2 teaspoon powdered ginger
- Salt and pepper

Method

1. Melt the butter in a heavy 4-quart pot over medium heat. When it foams, add the sliced garlic and onions and cook on medium-low heat for about 10 minutes, or until the onion is soft and translucent. Keep the heat low enough that the garlic doesn't brown; you want everything to sweat.
2. When the onions are soft, add the zucchini and cook until soft. Add the broth and bring to a simmer. Simmer at a low heat for about 45 minutes.
3. Let cool slightly, then blend with an immersion blender until creamy, or transfer to a standing blender to puree. Be very careful if you use the latter; only fill the blender half full with each batch, and hold the lid down tightly with a towel.
4. Taste and season with ginger, salt and pepper. Like most soups, this is significantly better after a night in the refrigerator to let the flavors meld.

Soothing Garlic Soup

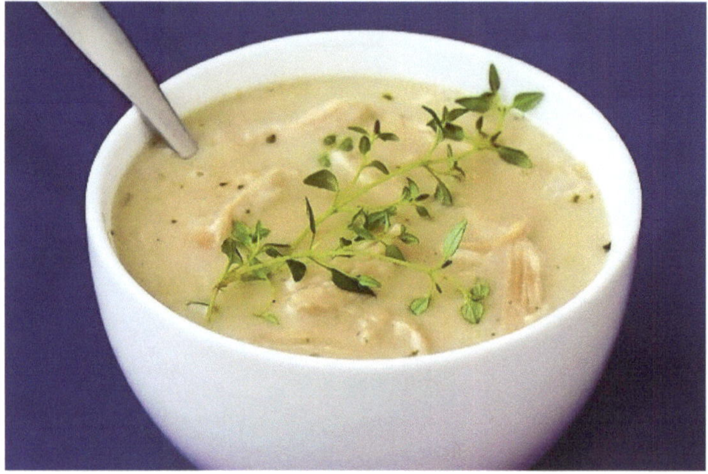

Serves: 6   Calories: 137

Preparation Time: 65 minutes

Ingredients

- 4-5 heads of garlic (45-50 cloves)
- 1/4 cup high quality olive oil
- 2 onions
- 4 tablespoons butter
- 1 quart of chicken broth
- 2 cups of coconut milk or other milk of choice
- 1 teaspoon dried thyme leaf or 2 teaspoons of fresh
- 1 teaspoon dried oregano leaf
- 1 teaspoon dried basil leaf
- 1/2 teaspoon salt
- 1/2 teaspoons black pepper
- 2 tablespoons fresh minced parsley leaf (optional)
- 1/4 cup chopped fresh chives (optional)
- 1 fresh lemon (for garnish)

Method

1. Preheat the oven to 350F/175C.
2. Cut the heads of garlic in half across the cloves but do not peel them.
3. Pour the olive oil into an oven safe dish and place the garlic head halves cut side down on the dish.Cover with an oven safe lid or foil.
4. Roast for 45 minutes to 1 hour or until garlic cloves are fragrant and starting to brown. To remove the garlic cloves, carefully pick up the shell of the garlic heads. The cloves should slightly stick to the pan, making peeling easy.

5. While garlic is roasting, melt butter in a large pot and add sliced onions. Saute over medium heat, stirring constantly until onions are translucent and golden. Add thyme, oregano, basil, salt and pepper and saute for 2 minutes.
6. When garlic is done roasting, add peeled cloves to the onion mixture in the pot.
7. Add chicken broth and bring to a simmer.
8. Simmer for 15 minutes.
9. Reduce heat to low and add coconut milk or other milk.
10. Using a stainless steel immersion blender, carefully blend the soup until smooth.
11. Serve warm.
12. Garnish with fresh parsley and chives and squeeze a lemon wedge over each bowl.

Tomato Soups

Tomato and Basil Soup

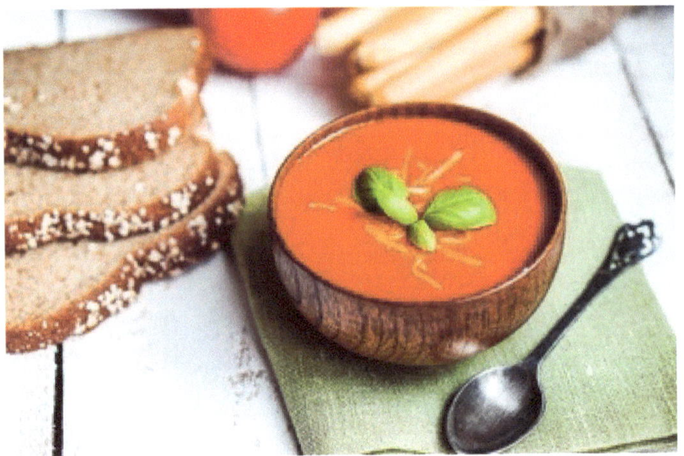

Serves: 4   Calories: Approx 750

Preparation Time: 25 minutes

Ingredients

- 2 tins tomatoes
- Approx 20 leaves of fresh basil
- 1 ½ cup chicken or vegetable stock
- 1 cup fresh cream
- 2 tbsp butter
- Pinch of sugar

Method

1. If the tomatoes are not already chopped, roughly chop them.
2. Add the tomatoes and stock to a saucepan and simmer for around ten minutes.
3. Roughly chop the basil and reserve a few pieces. Stir into the soup along with the sugar.
4. Slowly stir in the cream and butter, stirring gently, until the butter has melted.
5. Use the extra basil leaves as a garnish and serve immediately.

Hearty Tomato and Vegetable Soup

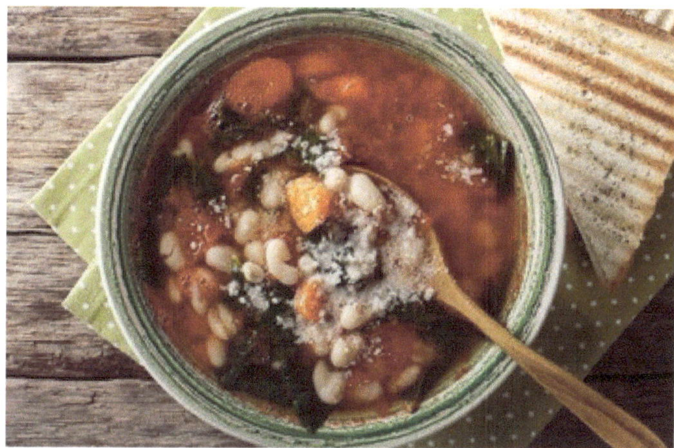

Serves: 4   Calories: Approx 600

Preparation Time: 60 minutes

Ingredients

- 1 tin tomatoes
- 1 cup chicken or vegetable stock
- 1 white onion
- 1 large potato
- 1 large carrot
- 2 sticks of celery
- ½ cup kidney or cannelloni beans
- 1 tsp dried oregano
- 1 tsp dried parsley
- 1 tbsp olive oil
- Pinch of salt
- Pinch of black pepper

Method

1. If the tomatoes are not already chopped, roughly chop them.
2. Dice the onion, potato, carrot and celery.
3. Heat the olive oil in a frying pan and cook the onions until soft and translucent. Set to one side.
4. Add the tomatoes and stock to a large saucepan and stir together.
5. Add the vegetables, herbs, salt and pepper to the soup and cook on a low heat for 40 minutes or until the potatoes and carrots are soft.
6. Serve hot and eat immediately.

Beef and Tomato Soup

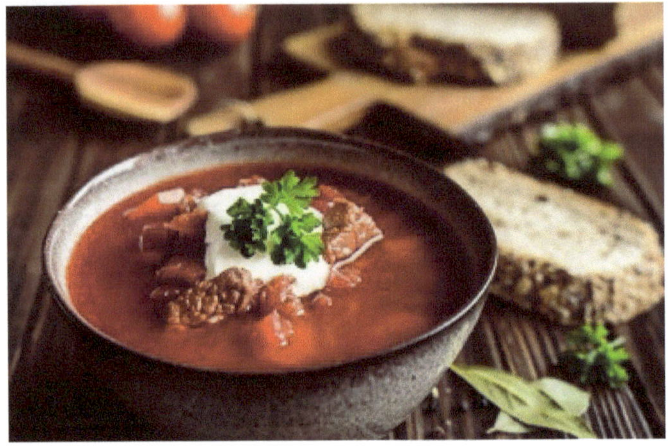

Serves: 6   Calories: Approx 1200

Preparation Time: 60-90 minutes

Ingredients

- 1 tin tomatoes
- 1 sirloin steak
- ½ white onion
- 1 green bell pepper
- 1 large potato
- 2 cups beef stock
- 1-2 tbsp olive oil or other cooking oil
- 2 tbsp tomato puree
- 1 tsp paprika
- Pinch of cayenne pepper
- Pinch of salt
- Pinch of black pepper
- 1 bay leaf

Method

1. If the tomatoes are not already chopped, roughly chop them.
2. Dice the steak.
3. Chop the onion, potato and green pepper.
4. Heat the oil in the bottom of a large pan and sauté the onion, green pepper and beef until the meat is thoroughly browned. Drain off any excess oil.
5. Add the stock, potato, seasoning and herbs.
6. Bring to the boil, then reduce heat and simmer for around 30 minutes, until the potato is soft.

7. Add the tomatoes and tomato puree. Stir thoroughly.
8. Cook for another 20-30 minutes or until the beef is tender and cooked through.
9. Remove the bay leaf before serving.

Spicy Fish Stew

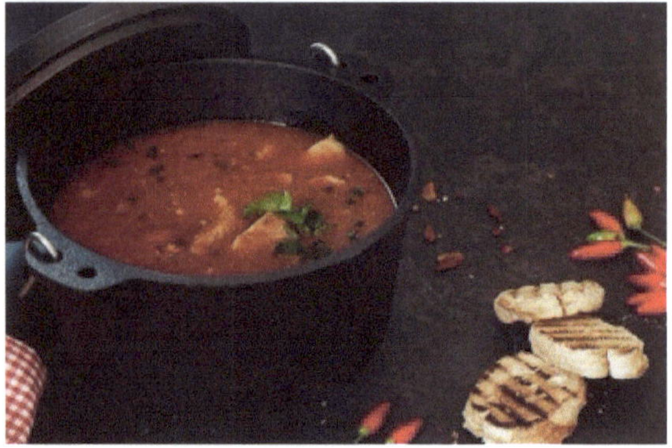

Serves: 4   Calories: Approx 550

Preparation Time: 20-30 minutes

Ingredients

- 1 tin tomatoes
- ½ white or yellow onion
- 1 clove garlic
- 1 tbsp olive oil
- 1-2 fillets of white fish
- ½ cup prawns/shrimp, cooked
- 1 tsp paprika
- 1 red chili pepper
- 1 tsp cilantro, chopped (optional)
- ½ cup water
- Pinch of salt

Method

1. If the tomatoes are not already chopped, roughly chop them.
2. Chop the onions and mince or finely chop the garlic.
3. Chop the fish into roughly 1-inch chunks.
4. De-seed and finely chop the chili pepper.
5. Heat the oil in a large saucepan. Add the onions, garlic and paprika and cook until the onions are soft.
6. Add the tomatoes and some water. Bring to the boil, then lower the heat.
7. Add the fish, salt and chili pepper and simmer for 10 minutes or until the fish is cooked almost through.
8. Stir in the prawns and cook for another 2 minutes or so.
9. Sprinkle with cilantro and serve hot with rice or crusty bread.

Gazpacho Soup

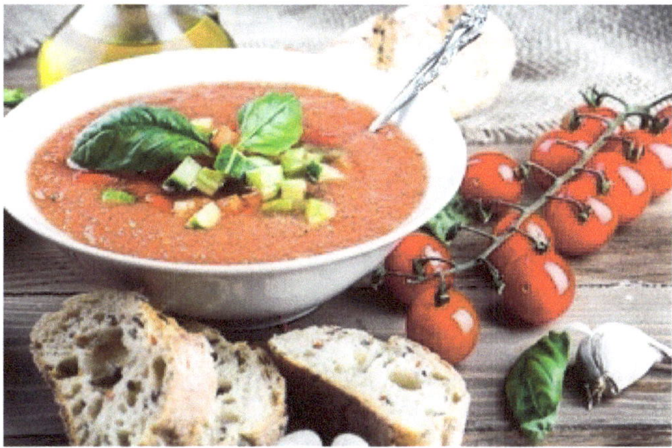

Serves: 4   Calories: Approx 600

Preparation Time: 20 minutes

Ingredients

- 2lb fresh, very ripe tomatoes
- 1 cucumber
- 2 green onions
- 1 red bell pepper
- 1 green bell pepper
- 1 garlic clove
- 1 piece of slightly stale French bread, about 4 inches long
- 2 tbsp sherry or red wine vinegar
- 1 tsp cumin (optional)
- 3 tbsp olive oil
- Pinch of salt

Method

1. Peel the cucumber and de-seed the peppers.
2. Roughly chop the cucumber, peppers, tomatoes, garlic and green onions, removing any tough stalks or cores from the tomatoes as you do so.
3. Soak the bread in cold water for around 10 minutes. When it's thoroughly soaked, pour the water away and squeeze as much water as possible from the bread.
4. Mix the vegetables, bread, vinegar, salt, cumin and 2 tbsp of olive oil in a blender until smooth.
5. Place the soup in the fridge to chill for at least an hour and serve cold, with a little olive oil drizzled over the top if you wish.

Egg Soups

Lemon Soup

An extremely flavorsome Greek soup. Serve with warm crusty bread with eggs for a delicious lunch.

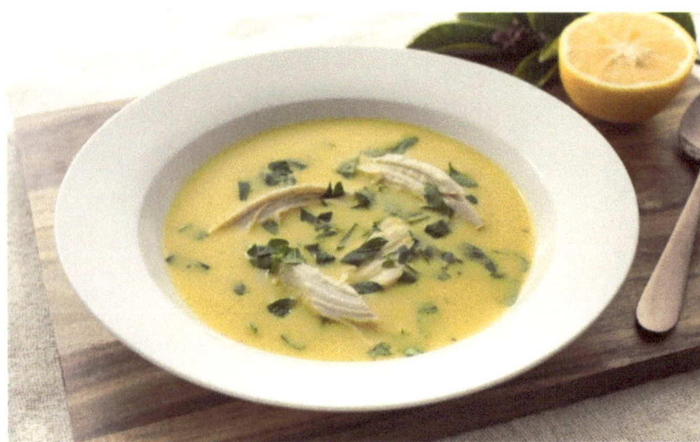

Serves: 6-8

Preparation Time: 1 hour 20 minutes

Ingredients

- 1 (35-40 ounce) fresh chicken
- 1 red onion (peeled)
- 5 cups cold water
- Salt and black pepper (for seasoning)
- 6-7 ounces plain rice
- 2 large eggs (at room temperature)
- Juice of 1 lemon

Method

1. Place the chicken in a large deep saucepan. Add the red onion, peeled but still whole. Add enough cold water to completely cover the bird. Season well with salt and pepper.
2. Place the saucepan over a high heat and bring to a boil. Reduce heat to medium and cover with a tightly fitting lid. Gently boil the chicken for approx. 60-70 minutes. (The chicken is cooked when the meat falls away from the carcass and juices run clear). Using a slatted spoon, skim off any surface foam from the water.
3. Remove the chicken from the pan and set aside.
4. Drain the broth and pour into a medium saucepan. Add the rice and season with salt and pepper. Bring to boil.

5. In the meantime, pull the chicken meat away from the bones and discard any skin. Cut the meat into bite size cubes.
6. Crack the 2 eggs into a clean large bowl. Whisk until foamy. Add the lemon juice and continue to whisk. Next, add a ladleful of the hot soup to the egg-juice mixture and whisk. Repeat this process until all the soup has been transferred to the bowl. The eggs should now be warm. Pour the mixture into the saucepan. Stir the soup, cover with a lid, and leave for 4-5 minutes.
7. Serve warm, sprinkled with the chicken cubes and seasoned with pepper.

Curry Egg Drop Soup

Egg drop soup, packed with vitamins and minerals, is a great cure-all for colds and sniffles.

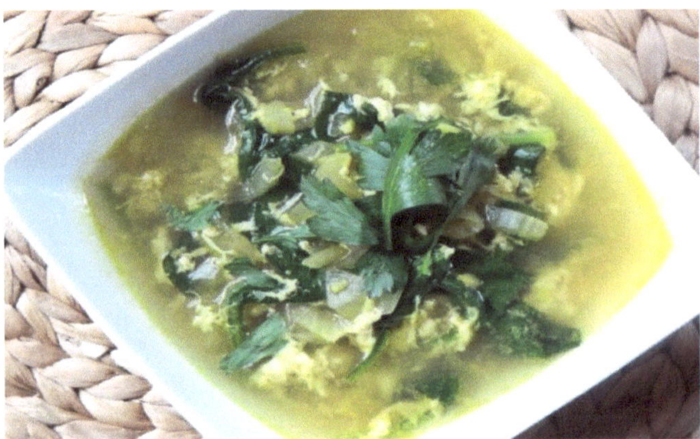

Serves: 2

Preparation Time: 15 minutes

Ingredients

- 1 tbsp. olive oil
- 1 yellow onion (finely chopped)
- 3 garlic cloves
- 1 small piece ginger (peeled, chopped)
- 1 tsp curry powder
- 4 cups vegetable stock
- salt and black pepper (to taste)
- 3 cups fresh spinach
- 2 medium eggs (beaten)
- fresh chopped parsley (to garnish)

Method

1. Heat the oil in a pot. When hot, add in the onions and sauté for 5 minutes, until softened.
2. Add in the garlic and ginger, sauté for another couple of minutes.
3. Sprinkle in the curry powder.
4. Pour in the vegetable stock, stir well and then season with salt and pepper. Turn the heat to a gentle simmer.
5. Toss in the spinach. After 30 seconds, take a wooden spoon and start to stir the soup, using large circular motions.
6. Continue to stir while you pour the beaten egg into the pot in a steady stream.
7. Ladle immediately into warm bowl and top with fresh parsley.

Italian Egg Soup

Although reminiscent of the classic Italian soup stracciatella, you won't find my recipe in an Italian cookbook. It's something I came up with that uses Italian ingredients in a way that satisfies me. This soup is thick, deeply flavorful, and easy to prepare, and it uses ingredients that I always have on hand.

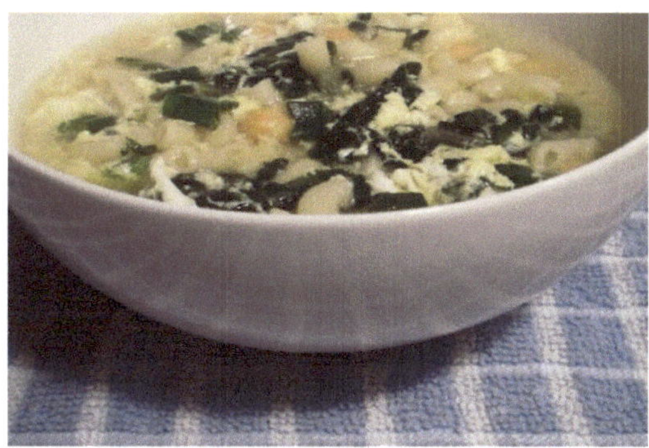

Serves: 6
Preparation Time: 30 minutes

Ingredients

- 6 ounces baby spinach
- 3 tablespoons extra-virgin olive oil
- ½ cup cubed pancetta
- 1 cup chopped onion
- 2 cloves garlic, minced
- ⅓ cup arborio rice
- 6 cups chicken broth
- ¼ cup grated Romano cheese
- 4 large eggs
- kosher salt
- freshly ground black pepper
- crushed hot red pepper flakes

Method

1. Wash the spinach (even if the bag says "washed"). Discard any mushy leaves. Heat the olive oil in a large pot. Toss in the pancetta and onion, and cook until the pancetta begins to brown and crisp and the onion softens and turns golden. Add the garlic and cook for a few minutes more.
2. Add the spinach to the pot and cook for about 2 minutes, until wilted. Stir in the rice.
3. Pour in the broth and bring to a simmer. Cover and cook at a low simmer for 20 minutes.

4. Using a fork, stir the cheese and eggs together in a bowl until well combined. Take the pot off the heat and, if desired, pour the soup into a serving tureen. Immediately stir in the egg-cheese mixture. It will cook when it hits the hot soup.
5. Taste and season with salt and pepper if necessary (this will depend on the saltiness of the broth).
6. Sprinkle with hot red pepper flakes.

Spanish Garlic Soup

This soup has the big flavors and full body that are perfect for a winter dinner. It is finished in the oven like French onion soup, but in this case, instead of melted cheese, there is an egg poached on the surface.

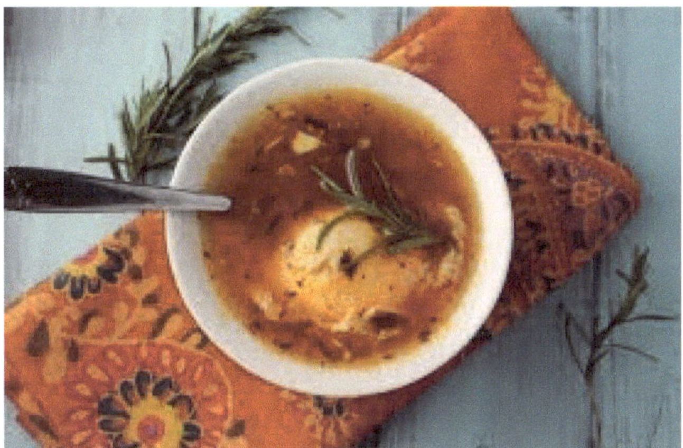

Serves: 4
Preparation Time: 25 minutes

Ingredients

- 3 tablespoons olive oil
- 6 cloves garlic, sliced
- 1 teaspoon sweet paprika
- ½ teaspoon cumin
- ⅛ teaspoon saffron
- 4 crusty bread slices
- chicken broth
- salt
- black pepper
- 4 eggs
- parsley

Method

1. Heat the olive oil in a large pot. Add the garlic and cook over low heat for about 10 minutes.
2. Add the ingredients.
3. Put the bread in the seasoned oil and toast on both sides.
4. Mix the broth in carefully over the bread.
5. Season with the salt and pepper. Bring the broth to a boil and then immediately lower the heat to a low simmer. If the soup boils too rapidly, the bread will break apart.

6. Preheat the oven to 400F / 205C. Put 4 ovenproof soup bowls on a baking sheet. Ladle the soup and a slice of bread into each bowl.
7. Crack an egg into each soup bowl. Slide the baking sheet into the oven (it's much easier than handling each bowl) and bake until the yolks are set, 8 to 10 minutes.
8. Sprinkle each serving with the cilantro.

Egg Drop Soup

This is a lighter, home-style recipe. It is very easy to prepare and makes a wonderful late-night supper when you come home tired and think there is nothing in the house.

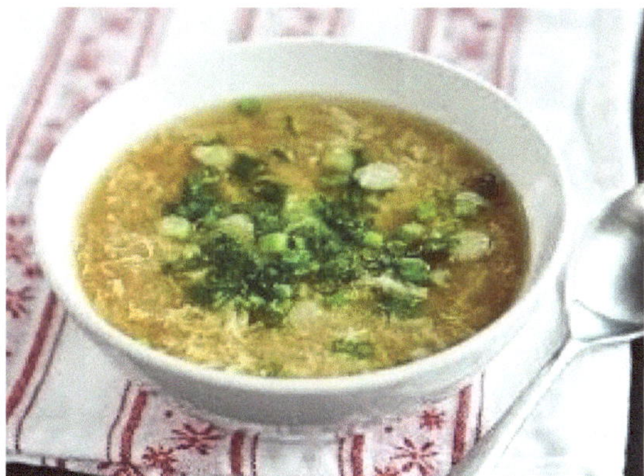

Serves: 4
Preparation Time: 20 minutes

Ingredients

- 4 cups chicken broth
- 2 slices peeled fresh ginger (about 1 by ⅛ inch)
- 2 cloves garlic, smashed and peeled
- 1 teaspoon kosher salt
- 2 large eggs
- 1 teaspoon dry sherry
- 2 scallions, sliced, using all the white and most of the green
- 2 tablespoons chopped fresh cilantro

Method

1. Bring the broth, ginger, and garlic to a boil in a large pot. Lower the heat and simmer gently for 5 minutes.
2. Discard the ginger and garlic. Stir in the salt. Lower the heat to a very low simmer.
3. In a small bowl, mix the eggs and sherry with a fork.
4. Pour the eggs into the soup in a slow, steady stream, swirling them into the soup. The eggs will set in strands.
5. Remove from the heat and stir in the scallions and cilantro.
6. Serve immediately. Enjoy!

Kids Soup Recipes
Simple Pumpkin Soup

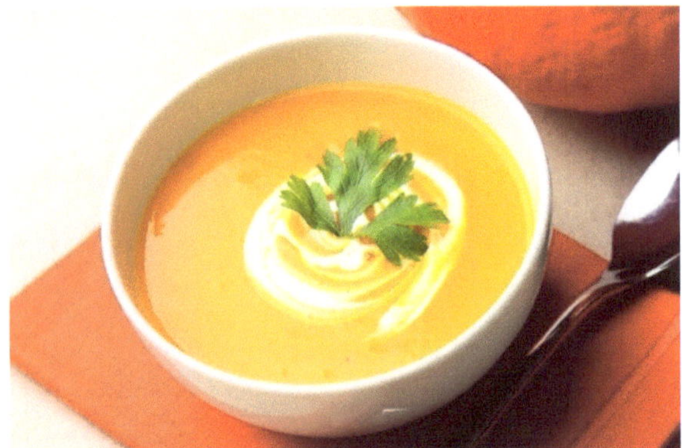

Serves: 8   Calories: approx. 180

Cook time: 30 minutes

Ingredients

- 1 butternut pumpkin, peeled de-seeded and cubed
- 1 large potato, peeled and cubed
- 1 large carrot, peeled and roughly chopped
- 1 onion, diced
- 2 tbsp. olive oil
- 4 tbsp. Massel chicken flavoured stock powder

Method

1. Heat oil in a pan and fry all vegetables until golden.
2. Add 2L boiling water to the pan and stir in stock powder.
3. Bring to the boil and simmer for 20 minutes until all vegetables are soft.
4. Using a stick mixer liquefy all the soup until it's nice and smooth.
5. Taste and season with salt and pepper accordingly.

Easy Homemade Soup

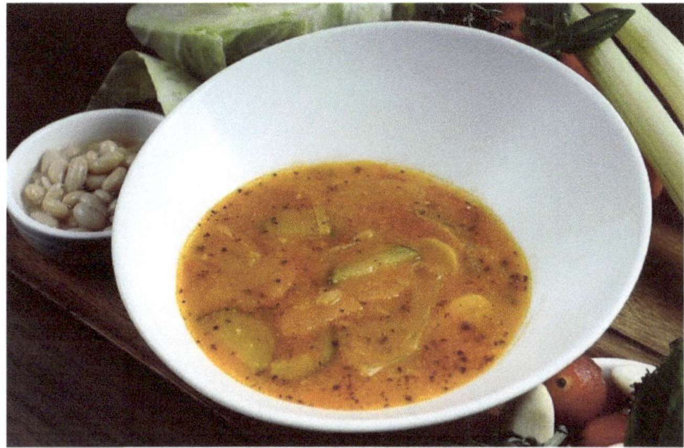

Serves: 4　Calories: approx. 100 per serving

Preparation Time: 20-30 minutes

Ingredients

- 1 onion
- 1 potato
- 1 small zucchini
- 1 stick celery
- 1 small leek
- 2 carrots
- 1 tbsp. oil
- 1 vegetable or chicken stock cube
- 1 tsp mixed herbs, dried or fresh

Method

1. Slice up the leek, carrot, zucchini and celery and dice the onion and potato. Older children should be able to do this themselves.
2. Add the oil to a frying pan and heat it up before adding the onions and zucchini. Fry for a few minutes until the onions soften and begin to turn golden.
3. Add the rest of the ingredients to a saucepan along with just enough water to cover them, and simmer gently until the vegetables are cooked through. Kids can check frequently to see how the vegetables are doing – the potatoes and carrots should be soft enough to poke a knife through.
4. Add the onions and zucchini to the soup and heat for another minute or two.
5. Serve with crusty bread.

The recipe for a joyful life!

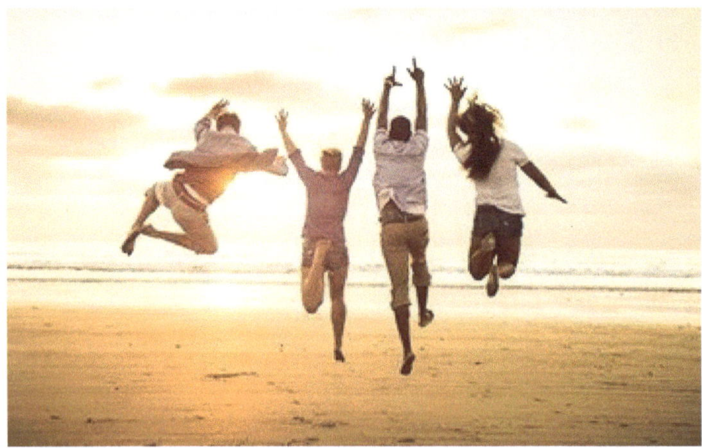

Serves: *all your family*

Cooking Time: *a few minutes every day*

Ingredients

- good mood
- positive thinking

Directions

- *Make small surprises for your loved ones*
- *Do charity work*
- *More often do your favorite thing*
- *Spend more time with children and the elderly*
- *Go in for sports*
- *Read books*
- *Learn the languages*
- *More walking*
- *Do exercises*
- *Throw away unnecessary things from home*
- *Plan an interesting weekend*
- *Take photos*
- *Smile more often*
- *Hug your loved ones*
- *Meditate*

www.ingramcontent.com/pod-product-compliance
Lightning Source LLC
Chambersburg PA
CBHW040141240726
48664CB00002B/567